S. A. ALLAZOV
I. S. ALLAZOV

CYSTIC NEOPLASMS OF THE SCROTAL ORGANS

S. A. ALLAZOV
I. S. ALLAZOV

CYSTIC NEOPLASMS OF THE SCROTAL ORGANS

Classification, simultaneous surgery along the Wesling line A monograph

ScienciaScripts

Imprint
Any brand names and product names mentioned in this book are subject to trademark, brand or patent protection and are trademarks or registered trademarks of their respective holders. The use of brand names, product names, common names, trade names, product descriptions etc. even without a particular marking in this work is in no way to be construed to mean that such names may be regarded as unrestricted in respect of trademark and brand protection legislation and could thus be used by anyone.

Cover image: www.ingimage.com

This book is a translation from the original published under ISBN 978-620-8-22390-8.

Publisher:
Sciencia Scripts
is a trademark of
Dodo Books Indian Ocean Ltd. and OmniScriptum S.R.L publishing group

120 High Road, East Finchley, London, N2 9ED, United Kingdom
Str. Armeneasca 28/1, office 1, Chisinau MD-2012, Republic of Moldova, Europe
Managing Directors: Ieva Konstantinova, Victoria Ursu
info@omniscriptum.com

Printed at: see last page
ISBN: 978-620-8-35288-2

MINISTRY OF HEALTH OF THE REPUBLIC OF UZBEKISTAN
SAMARKAND STATE MEDICAL UNIVERSITY

ALLAZOV S.A., ALLAZOV I.S.

CYSTIC NEOPLASMS OF THE SCROTAL ORGANS (CLASSIFICATION, SIMULTANEOUS SURGERY ALONG THE WESLING LINE)

MONOGRAPH

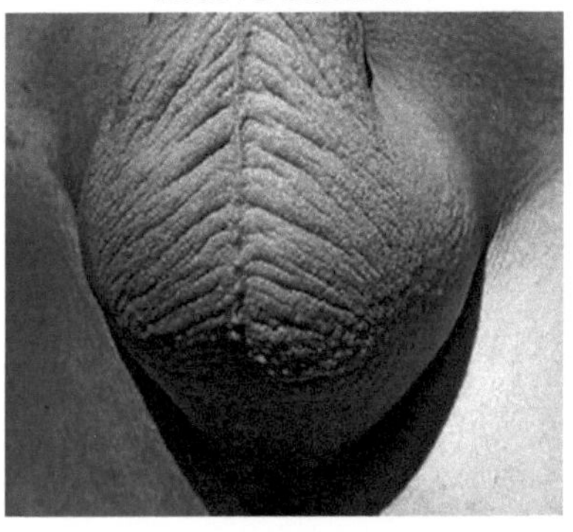

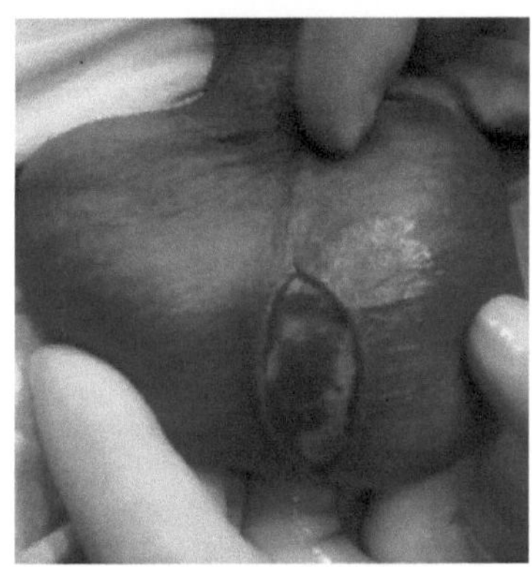

SAMARKAND 2024

ALLAZOV S.A., ALLAZOV I.S. CYSTIC NEOPLASMS OF THE SCROTAL ORGANS (CLASSIFICATION, SIMULTANEOUS SURGERY) ON THE WESLING LINE)

REVIEWERS:

SHERBEKOV U.A. HEAD OF THE DEPARTMENT OF GENERALSURGERY OF SAMSMU, DOCTOR OF MEDICAL SCIENCES, ASSOCIATE PROFESSOR.

KOBILOV E.E. HEAD OF THE DEPARTMENT OF ECOLOGY ANDLIFE SAFETY OFSAMSU NAMED AFTER SHAROF RASHIDOV, DR.M.SC., PROF.

FOR UROLOGISTS, ANDROLOGISTS, ONCOUROLOGISTS, PHYSICIANS OF ALLIED SPECIALITIES, CLINICAL RESIDENTS, AND MASTER'S RESIDENTS.

TABLE OF CONTENTS

SUMMARY

The monograph is devoted to the problem of using a median incision along the Wessling line for simultaneous simultaneous simultaneous performance of simultaneous surgical intervention on the organs of both halves of the scrotum (testicular appendage cyst, testicular hydrocele, testicular cyst and hydrocele, operations on both testicles during -pulp-or orchiectomy for prostate cancer, etc.). The results of simultaneous operations on the scrotal organs along the Wessling line have cosmetic advantages, convenience of operative access, cost-effectiveness and reduction of the duration of the operation itself.

INTRODUCTION

Relevance. Common diseases of the scrotal organs are malformations (separation of the middle line of the sacs, aplasia, hypoplasia and ectopia of the testicles, cryptorchidism), testicular torsion, trauma, inflammatory diseases (epididymitis, orchitis, tuberculosis of the appendage and testis, brucellosis orchitis), testicular hydrocele, haematocele, funiculocele, spermatocele, varicocele, tumours of the testis and its appendage.(Batirov B.A.,Gafarov R.R.,2024).In operations for the above-mentioned conditions, if unilateral, scrotal skin incisions are usually made on the corresponding side of the disease or lesion. At the same time, difficulties and difficulties arise in cases of bilateral processes requiring surgical intervention in both halves of the scrotum. The problem of bilateral surgical intervention on both healthy testicles (orch-, pulpectomy) in prostate cancer is of particular importance. (Vozianov S.O., Ishmuradov B.T. 2023). Still many make incisions on both sides of the scrotum, which is traumatic and non-cosmetic in one way or another.In this question, one would have to be aware of the presence of the mid scrotal suture (Wesling's line), which is actually an extension of the white line of the abdomen on the scrotum. An incision along this line is considered appropriate for access to both halves of the scrotum and its organs, a so-called simultaneous operation for various diseases. (Allazav I.S. 2024). It should be noted that daily introduction of simultaneous operations (CO) in surgical, including urological, practice will become, firstly, one of the most important successes of medicine; secondly, a stimulus for health care development; thirdly, it will facilitate treatment of patients with several diseases of surgical and urological profile. But despite such a high need for CRM according to this World Health Organisation [WHO] 25-30% (1995) of those seeking surgical care; in 2.8-63%), the latter are performed only in 1.5-6.0% of cases (Lebedeva E.A., 2010; Baigazakov A. T., 2015 ; Temurbulatov V.M. et al., 2016; Murodov A.I., 2017). Before 1980-1990s. The majority of specialists did not accept CRM, which is related to the predominance of open interventions under less than perfect anaesthesia and surgical equipment. Intervention "in one surgical session" of two surgical technologies was usually accompanied by an increase in traumatic access and the risk of anaesthetic complications, especially in cases of prolonged anaesthesia. Modern high-precision minimally invasive laparoscopic methods of treatment have contributed to the reduction of traumatic access, blood loss, elimination of infection. At the same time, many consider inexpedient to perform laparoscopic CRM in patients whose objective status corresponds to ASA-II or ASA-III due to the increase of elderly people belonging to this category (Lyulko A.A. et al., 2015; Serdyukova M.A. et al., 2017; Gaar E.V., 2017; Gillen S. et al., 2010; Silverstein A. et al., 2016). At the same time, deterioration of organ functions aggravates surgical stress and elderly patients after undergone surgical interventions become more susceptible to perioperative diseases (Temurbulatov V.M. et al., 2016; Gerbali O.Y., 2019). The factors limiting the use of CRM also include the following points: a. the need for prolonged maintenance of carboxyperitoneum during laparoscopic surgeries; b. increased duration of surgical intervention. These causative factors contribute to the increase in the development of thrombophlebitis of the lower limb veins, hypoventilation of the lungs due to the non-physiological mechanism of breathing, thromboembolic complications due to decreased blood flow velocity, disorders of the mechanisms of heart rhythm regulation, etc. (Bunatyan A.A., Mizikov V.M., 2011; Medvdev V.L., 2015; Kotelnikova L.P., 2015, Kogan M.I. et al., 2021).But in any case, at this time, according to most authors, CRMs have a great perspective (PushkarD.Y., 2010; Semyonov V.V., Kurigin Al.A., 2014; Bunatyan D.A., 2016; Satkaeva A.J., 2016; Gerbeli O.Y., 2019). The advantages of CRM in comparison with MO are: 1. Safe elimination of a disease state in the process of only one intervention; 2 . Reduction of treatment time 3. Exclusion of the probability of exacerbation of concomitant disease in the future; 4. Reduction of the need for repeated surgery with the next preoperative examination;5.anaesthesiological load, emotional experience of the patient, etc. In surgical treatment of various combined diseases of abdominal cavity, retroperitoneal space and pelvic cavity (simultaneous interventions for cholelithiasis and kidney cysts, inguinal hernia and varicocele on the left side, inguinal hernia and congenital cryptorchidism simultaneous radical posterior prostatectomy and inguinal hernia plasty) encouraging results were obtained, although S. V. Papova and co-authors (2022), the share of CO from all interventions was 8, 39 %, and the share of MO - 8, 39 %.V. Papova et al. (2022), the proportion of CO from all interventions was 8, 39 %, and the proportion of MO was 91, 61 %. At the same time, there are few publications devoted to simultaneous interventions and insufficient development of the CRM problem in general, the need for further research is confirmed (PushkarD.Yu., 2010; Semyonov V.V., Kurigin Al.A., 2014, 2017; Satkaeva A.J., 2016; Muradov A.I., 2017; Gerbeli O.Y., 2019).

CHAPTER I

SURGICAL ACCESSES FOR SCROTAL OPERATIONS
(literature review)

As is known, frequent diseases of the external genital organs in men are malformations (midline separation of the sacs, underdevelopment, aplasia, hypoplasia and ectopia of the testicles, cryptorchidism) (Kogan M.I.,2021), testicular torsion (Kalinina S.N., et al.,2019), injuries (Nazarov T.H., et al, 2020), inflammatory diseases (Voronik G.M., 2008; Bashembiev H.M., et al., 2010; Prokhorov A.V., 2015, 2016) (epididymitis, orchitis, tuberculosis of the appendage and testis, brucellosis orchitis), testicular hydrocele, haematocele, funiculocele, spermatocele, varicocele (Kapto A.A., 2016; Broz M.P. etal., 2013; Iacona F. etal., 2014; Rogue M. etal., 2018), tumours of the testis and its appendage. In operations for the above conditions, if unilateral, scrotal skin incisions are usually made on the corresponding side of the disease or lesion. Although the best possible access should be chosen when the pathology is unilateral. At the same time, difficulties and difficulties arise in cases of bilateral process, requiring surgical intervention in both halves of the scrotum. (Allazov S.A., Allazov I.S., 2023). Bilateral surgical interventions on both testicles (orch-, pulpectomy) in prostate cancer are also problematic. (Vozianov S.O., Ishmuradov B.T., 2023). Until now, many still make incisions on both lateral surfaces of the scrotum, which is somehow traumatic and non-cosmetic.

In this matter, we should use the midline suture of the scrotum (Wesling's line), which is actually an extension of the white line of the abdomen to the scrotum (Leshenko I.G. et al., 2011; Allazov S.A. et al., 2015, 2019).

It is considered reasonable to make an incision along this line in order to access both halves of the scrotum and its organs, the so-called simultaneous operation in case of various diseases through a single incision and under one and lower napposis (S.A. Allazov. et al., 2018).Quite often in clinical practice, there are cases of combined pathologies of the organs of both halves of the scrotum, in connection with which there are indications for performing simultaneous operations. Simultaneous operations are performed on different organs through a single access. In contrast to simultaneous multi-organ operations, multi-organ operations are performed on different organs at the same time alternately through different accesses, here for different operations are performed through a single access to perform simultaneous operations on organs of both halves of the scrotum, the most convenient is an incision along the midline of the scrotum (raphe scroti), which is called after the name of the scientist who first described it - Wesling's line Study of the possibilities of surgical treatment of diseases of organs of one or both halves of the scrotum by means of transmoshonojejunal access along the Wesling's line. The problem is particularly acute with regard to simultaneous operations on both apparently healthy testicles (bilateral pulpectomy for prostate cancer) (Keshishev N.G., et al. 2010). Bilateral pulpectomy or orchiectomy is still widely used in the copulmonary treatment of cancer. This disease is a complex problem of modern medicine, being the most frequent pathology among tumours of the urogenital system (Chissov V.I. et al. 2009; 2013; Matveev B.P. 2011). The growth of prostate cancer morbidity reaches 3% per year. Many elderly men have comorbidities that preclude radical surgery. Radiation therapy or its combination with hormone therapy are alternative methods. Among all hormone-dependent tumours, RPZ is the most sensitive to hormonal effects (Glbochko P.V. et al., 2014). About 70 years ago it was established that testosterone is the main hormone regulating the mitotic activity of PG cells. For the first time, the dependence of PG tumour cells on the level of testosterone in blood serum In his study of Huggins etal. in 1941, he showed that the growth and development of both normal and malignant PG cells depends on serum testosterone concentration. He proved that the growth and development of both normal and malignant PG cells depends on serum testosterone concentration, and demonstrated the efficacy of surgical castration and estrogen therapy in the progression of metastatic RPF. After their seminal studies, hormone therapy (HT) has become the mainstay of treatment for patients with advanced RPF (M1) as well as patients with regional lymph node involvement (N+) due to the peculiarities of the clinical course of 60 to 80% of RPF patients at. The growth, proliferation and development of PJ cells are largely dependent on androgens. Testosterone is not directly the cause of the occurrence of AD, but plays an essential role in regulating the mechanism of growth and development of tumour cells. The essence of therapeutic measures is to maximally reduce the concentration of endogenous testosterone - the so-called androgen blockade. Inhibition or reduction of the concentration of the cytoplasmic androgen receptor. Orchidectomy is an effective method of reducing the main biological active androgen, testosterone, in the blood, but has no effect on the production of adrenal androgens. Surgical castration is still considered to be ais the "gold standard" for antiandrogen therapy (Allazov S.A., 2021). Removal of the testes, which are the main source of androgens, leads to a significant decrease in testosterone levels and causes a hypogonadal state, although a small level of testosterone remains (castration level). Bilateral orchiectomy is an easily performed surgical procedure, which is performed and

Leshenko I.G. et al, (Medvedov 2015., Allazov S.A. et al, 2019; Allazov S.A., Gafarov,2021 under local anaesthesia and has virtually no complications. It is a fast (less than 12 hours) way to achieve castration testosterone levels. The main disadvantage of the method is the negative psychological effect. The irreversibility of surgical castration is an obstacle to intermittent therapy. While antiandrogenic therapy is palliative in its effectiveness, it can stop the growth of cancer cells, change the biological potential of the tumour, stop the processes of further metastasis, "reduce" the stage of the tumour process. According to N.L. Lopatkin (2007), a part of patients seeking medical help for urological complications already have a verified diagnosis of cancer, and may have received any type of treatment. In order to obtain optimal results, even if temporary, it is necessary to individualise treatment to the maximum extent possible, taking into account concomitant pathology (atherosclerosis, CHD, hypertension, diabetes mellitus, etc.). The problem of palliative care in oncourology requires a multifaceted approach. The term "palliative" comes from the Latin "pallium", meaning "mask" or "cloak". This defines what palliative care is essentially: palliation - hiding the manifestations of an incurable disease and/or providing a cloak-cover to protect those left "out in the cold, unprotected". As defined by WHO (2002), palliative care is a branch of medical and social action that aims to improve the quality of life of incurable patients and their families by preventing and alleviating their suffering through early detection, careful assessment and management of pain and other symptoms: physical, psychological and spiritual. In modern oncology, it is necessary to assess treatment outcomes not only by survival and life expectancy criteria or tumour response to treatment, but also by specific measures of quality of life. In fact, even palliative treatment includes rehabilitation, the aim of which is to help patients achieve and maintain their maximum physical, psychological, social and spiritual potential, however limited these may be as a result of disease progression. The relevance of the introduction of endovideosurgical technologies in one-stage (simultaneous) operations is due to the increasing number of patients with combined surgical diseases. According to WHO data, almost 63% of patients arriving to a surgical hospital need one-stage operations. Prior to the introduction of endovideosurgical technologies, it was believed that the performance of one-stage operations was essentially increases surgical aggression, leads to an increase in the number of intra- and postoperative complications and worsens the results of surgical treatment, especially when it is necessary to use two surgical accesses (Leshchenko I.G. et al., 2011;2012). With the development of endovideosurgical technique, the question arose about the possibility of expanding the indications for one-stage operations. This was due to the main advantage of laparo-peak interventions - minimal trauma access, which found application in the performance of one-stage operations in surgery and gynaecology (Muslimov Sh.T. 2013;. As for one-stage operations for combined urological diseases or their combination with diseases of abdominal cavity organs, they are not widely covered in the available literature (Popov O.V. et al., 2022). In this connection it is reasonable to consider the most frequently occurring variants of combinations of urological diseases, as well as combinations of urological and surgical pathologies, additional arguments "for" and "against" one-stage operations in these combinations. One of the most common surgical diseases is cholelithiasis (GI). In Russia, the annual incidence of LCDD averages 5-6 per 1000 population per year, i.e., about 1 million people per year Lisov N.A. et al., 2016 Partly the wide prevalence is explained by the high frequency of combination of LCDD with diseases of abdominal cavity organs, gynaecological and urological pathology. In addition, there are common pathogenetic links between cholelithiasis and various urological diseases such as urolithiasis [4-13] and nephroptosis [14-16]. There are strong clinical arguments in favour of the simultaneous treatment of GI and coexisting urological diseases. Thus, combined cholecystectomy excludes the possibility of complications of GI in the postoperative period. In modern literature there are many descriptions of this complication, which required cholecystectomy in the immediate postoperative period[17-25]. Such a complication is extremely unfavourable: postoperative cholecystitis is characterised by a more severe course, and the results of treatment are much worse than in uncomplicated cholecystitis Ventral hernias are often combined with diseases of the abdominal cavity and urinary system. According to different data [28, 29], hernias are present in almost 3-4% of the whole population, in 14-25% of patients with hernias one combined disease or more is found, causing the need for active surgical intervention. An example of the common pathogenesis of ventral hernias with diseases of the urinary system are prostate diseases - benign hyperplasia (BPH) or cancer (BP), leading to infravesical obstruction and, accordingly, constant pushing during urination. The resulting increase in intra-abdominal pressure can lead to both progression of existing hernias and the appearance of new ones [8, 28, 30, 31]. The question of the necessity of combined treatment is quite acute in these cases for the following reasons. Postponement of hernia intervention is dangerous with the development of complications in the early postoperative period, because against the background of probable intestinal paresis there is a persistent increase in intra-abdominal pressure. Hernia impingement in the early postoperative period puts the patient in an extremely unfavourable situation: there is a need for emergency re-intervention immediately after the first operation against the background of depletion of reserve systems of the body.In a staged approach to the treatment of combined diseases of the urinary system and hernias, there is a risk of hernia progression [31-34], whereas a one-stage operation for hernia and adenoma or prostate or RP avoids both acute urinary retention and hernia impingement in the postoperative period [28, 35]. The presence of an unoperated or fixed hernia is considered a contraindication to performing laparoscopic interventions [36], as the application of a carboxyperitoneum may lead to hernia impingement in the postoperative period. In this situation, there are two alternatives: either one-stage laparoscopic surgery, or abandoning the laparoscopic access and performing the operation using the traditional open method. In the latter case, the intestinal paresis arising after isolated surgery due to persistent increase in intra-abdominal pressure also can lead to hernia progression and impingement [37], and open combined surgery often has to be performed from two accesses, which may worsen the postoperative period due to purulent-septic complications [1].Combined urological diseases are a common problem. Close functional connection of the urinary system organs leads to the emergence and development of complications in the form of lesions of the second and more organs in the case of pathology of one. Thus, urolithiasis is bilateral, according to different data [8, 29, 38], in 15-30%. Most often it is observed in the formation of large and coral-like stones, which is associated with the specific influence of pathogenesis factors on both kidneys (for example, in hyperparathyroidism). Bilateral renal lesions such as nephroptosis (8-23%), hydronephrosis (4.8-17%), and solitary renal cysts (9%) are common in clinical practice. Bilateral renal tumours are increasingly detected [8, 29].The literature describes cases and small series of endovideosurgical combined interventions for the combination of cholelithiasis and urinary system organs [39, 40], ventral hernia and urological pathology [41-43], combined diseases of urogenital apparatus [44-48]. All authors come to the opinion that it is technically possible to perform these interventions, emphasise their safety and effectiveness [39, 44-56], while noting the lack of data in the literature on classification, indications and contra-indications, peculiarities of these operations [16, 21, 37]. The latter circumstance makes it necessary to study this issue in more depth. In 1971, Professor A. Shelly isolated native LHRH and in 1977 received the Nobel Prize for his work on brain peptide hormones. This led to the development of LHRH agonist therapy as a method of medically induced castration. Currently, HT hormone therapy is the mainstay of treatment for locally advanced cancer. The choice of type and timing of hormone therapy (HT) is based on the judgement of the physician and the informed consent of the patient. Androgen deprivation (AD) is effective in more than 90 per cent of patients (including advanced stages of BPH). The role of neoadjuvant and adjuvant hormonal therapy in addition to local surgical or radiotherapy has been reported, and studies on alternative regimens of hormonal therapy (intermittent therapy) are underway. The main options for androgen deprivation are:

1.Medical castration

2.Surgical castration

3.Flare blockade + medical castration

4.Antiandrogen monotherapy

5.Antiandrogens + 5-alpha reductase inhibitors

6.Combined androgen deprivation

7.Intermittent androgen deprivation

8.Triplet drug therapy

Neoadjuvant therapy was used to reduce the incidence of positive surgical margins and possibly improve the outcome of radical prostatectomy. Seven randomised trials have demonstrated that neoadjuvant therapy reduces the incidence of positive surgical margins for clinically localised stage; data for locally advanced disease are less conclusive. The aim of adjuvant therapy is to cases and better cancer-specific survival compared with those who received delayed treatment (62va 71%;p < 0.001). These results are similar to those obtained in patients with metastatic prostate cancer.Several studies have investigated intermittent hormonal blockade to evaluate the reduction of side effects following AD, the improvement of quality of life in advanced process and the delay in the development of hormonal refractoriness [10]. These studies were based on the assumption that intermittent BP can lead to a long-term decrease in serum testosterone levels. Randomised trials are currently underway to determine the effects of intermittent therapy. Therapy on survival.

CHAPTER II

MATERIAL AND METHODS RESEARCH

II.1 General characterisation of the clinical material

The monograph is based on clinical analysis of the results of urological care in 50 patients. Clinical examination, surgical treatment and postoperative follow-up of patients were carried out on the basis of the Department of Urology, SamSMU and Sam. RSCEMP (Director - Candidate of Medical Sciences Yangiev B.A.) for 2021-2024.
The mean age of the patients was 48.4±1.6 years (range 30-90 years).

Patients were divided into two single-digit groups:

1- group -30 patients with surgical access through the Wesling line.

2- group - 20 patients with traditional access.

The absolute number of all surgical interventions in general, all CRMs and the corresponding separately performed MIs performed routinely during the period under review was respectively, i.e. the share of CRMs from all interventions performed during that period was 8.39%, the share of mono-operations was 91.61%.
It should be noted that diagnostic and treatment standards should be integrated primarily by urologists, as well as allied specialists (Allazov S.A., 2010; Allazov S.A. et al., 2011).
The following perioperative parameters were analysed in each case: duration of the operation, volume of intraoperative blood loss (IOB); duration of MF drainage with urethral catheter, frequency of infectious and inflammatory complications (IIC) of the genitourinary system in the immediate postoperative period, duration of hospital stay in the postoperative period, duration of CMA and ETN induction, duration of patients' awakening (this parameter was considered only in those cases when the patient was not awake). Statistical analysis of the obtained data was performed by means of two-sample two-tailed t-test (computer application software package Statistica,10.0). Differences were considered significant at <0.05. Statistical processing was performed by using the << IBM SPSS Statistics >> (version 23, Russian language) programme with the << Comparison of averages >> function (analysis of mean comparison T-test for paired samples.

The diagnosis of RPV is based on the combined use of the following components:

- prostate-specific antigen (PSA) test;
- Finger rectal examination (FRE);
- transrectal puncture biopsy of the prostate gland under the control of transrectal ultrasound.The final diagnosis is established on the basis of the data of the puncture biopsy of the prostate gland.
-

II.2 Research Methods.

Examination of the studied patients selected in the main and control groups was carried out according to a unified algorithm (protocol of management), the basis of which and the most important method was colour and pulse-wave echo-dopplerography.

The algorithm of patient management consistently included: collection of complaints, clarification of medical and life history, objective examination of the patient in ortho- and clinostasis with performance of functional tests - Valsalva and Ivanissevich, general blood analysis (coagulation determination), Coagulogram, ejaculate analysis, , testicular ultrasound and scrotal echo-dopplerography, testiculometry, orchidoaxillothermometry ureteral catheterisation and excretory urography.

Also, all other patients underwent transabdominal ultrasound examination with colour Doppler mapping of the venous systems of the left kidney. The structural ultrasonographic examination of the kidneys and ultrasonographic examination of the scrotal organs were performed in some patients, as indicated.

Methods of physical examination and performance of functional tests

Next, the patient's scrotal organs were examined and palpated, standing and lying in a warm room to reduce the effect of the cremasteric reflex, at rest and when pushing. These methods were used to establish the clinical diagnosis of varicocele. In the vertical position of the patient both seminal canals were visually examined in order to detect the difference in their size, and on palpation the degree of prolapse of the worm-like dilated veins of the seminal canal relative to the level of the testicles according to Nicheporenko. The presence of any signs of testicular atrophy (flabbiness of tissue, reduction in size) was noted.

Functional tests and determination of the degree of varicocele. All patients under study underwent functional tests - Ivanissevich, "coughing jerk", Valsalva test. The "coughing jerk" test (a variant of the symptom of P. Zablotsky, 1848) was performed during palpation of the spermatic cord on both sides. Its mechanism is associated with the transmission of increased intra-abdominal pressure to the dilated veins of the bunched plexus, in healthy people this impulse is not determined (the test is negative). Ivanissevich's test (Segond R. 1885) was performed in all patients. In a patient in clinostasis, the spermatic cord at the level of the external ring of the inguinal canal was pressed against the brow bone, then without stopping the pressing of the spermatic cord, the patient was transferred to orthostasis. The degree of vein filling with blood was assessed. The absence of filling during compression and filling of the plexus after stopping the pressure on the spermatic cord indicated a positive test. The presence of slow filling of the plexus with blood at continued compression indicated possible venous discharge into the iliac vein system, which required further echo-Doppler confirmation. Detection of a marked varicocele persisting in ortho- and clinostasis during physical examination allowed us to assume its secondary (symptomatic) nature and the presence of persistent venous hypertension. Such patients (27 patients) were excluded from the study and referred to a vascular surgeon for consultation and treatment. It was only when it was necessary to diagnose varicocele for surgical treatment that the modified Valsalva test was used. The fundamental difference is that Valsalva proposed the technique of forced exhalation with the mouth and nostrils (strongly closed), and in the diagnosis of varicocele the patient is offered to hold his breath during inhalation, and - to push [Lopatkin N. A. et al., 1985]. In this case, the increase in the volume of the seminal canal veins indicates the presence of varicocele. In our studies, this test was used mainly in ultrasound of the scrotal organs with Doppler ultrasound. At objective examination, almost all patients appeared healthy and strong. No noticeable deviations from the norm were found in the organs of the thoracic and abdominal cavity, as well as in the organs of the urinary system.

II.2.2 Determination of testicular size (orchidometry)

The orchidometer (or testiculometer Prader) is a measuring device that is designed for comparative assessment of testicular volume. The device was proposed in 1966 by Andrea Prader, an endocrinologist from Switzerland. The orchidometer consists of a chain of twelve numbered wooden or plastic beads that increase in size from 1 to 25 millilitres (Fig.1a). The pellets of the orchidometer are compared to the patient's testicles and the volume is read from the bead that is most appropriately sized.(Fig 1b). The size during prepubertal period is 1-3 ml, during puberty it is 4 ml and above, and in adults it is 12 to 25 ml.In the case of varicocele, it is necessary to establish the fact of secondary hypogonadism, i.e. a reduction in the size of the testis on the affected side.

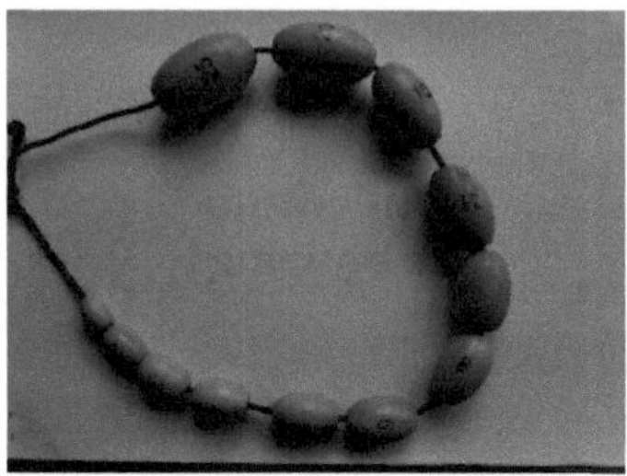

Figure 1a. Prader's testiculometer

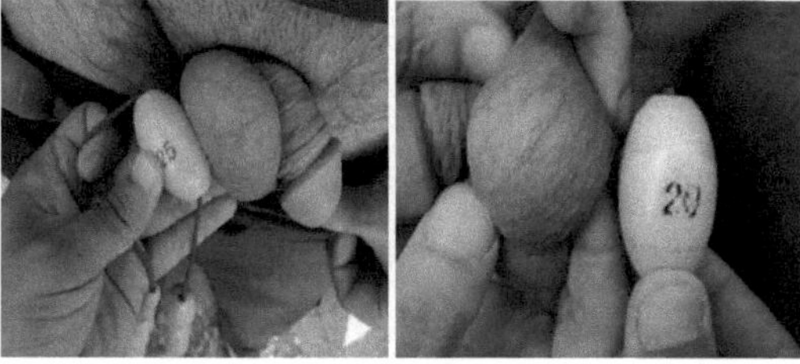

Fig. 1b. Orchidometry of the right and left testis.

Orchidoaxillothermometry.

Thermometry is a routine method and reflects the state of testicular blood flow through the scrotal skin. We used a mercury medical thermometer for all patients, and the examination was carried out in rooms at room temperature (+24 ±2°). Before the examination, the patient should be undressed for 10 - 15 min to adapt to the ambient temperature. Thermometry was performed on both sides in the supine position and differences in temperature values were detected. In case of varicocele the temperature difference varied from 1.0 to 3.0° C, after surgery this gradient disappeared. This is our method of Comparative Multilocal Orchidothermometry, which is an alternative to 2 methods, electronic thermometry and non-contact thermometry. infrared thermography of the scrotum in the diagnosis of varicocele proposed by Kapto A.A. et al. (2018).

Both methods establish the fact of scrotal hyperthermia in varicocele, which varies greatly in its acute complications. Here, a medical thermometer, comparatively measures the temperature of both halves of the scrotum and axillary regions.(Fig.2).

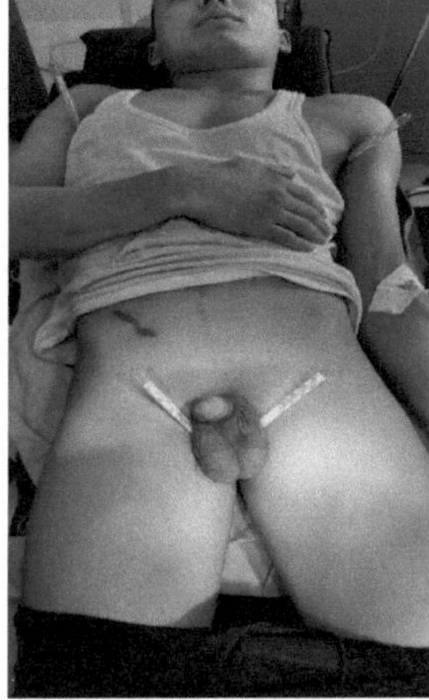

Figure 2. Orchidaxillothermometry.

Coagulogram - indicators of blood haemostasis:

Haemostasis is a physiological system of the body, the purpose of which is to keep the blood in a liquid state, this system consists of 3 components: clotting, anti-clotting and fibrinolytic. If the balance between them is disturbed, hyper or hypo coagulopathies develop. Standards coagulogram indicators have different variants, here is one of them. In the general blood analysis has the value of "Time of blood coagulation according to Sukharev" which is considered normal: the beginning of fibrinogenesis from 30 to 120 seconds, the end from 3 to 5 minutes. The following table is considered to be a more detailed interpretation of the haemostasis system.(Table 1).

Table1. Coagulogram parameters

№	Indicators	Unitsв norm
1	Prothrombin index	more than 80 per cent
2	Plasma recalcification time	60-120 c
3	Thrombotest	IV-V degrees
4	Fibrinogen	5,9-11,7 μmol/L
5	Fibrinogen B	negative
6	Fibrinolytic activity	183-263 min
7	Plasma tolerance to heparin	3-6 (7-11) min.
8	Lee-White time	5-10 min
9	Duration of bleeding on Duke.	up to 4 min
10	Blood clot retraction	44-65%

scrotal ultrasound

According to ultrasound, testicular volume in our patients with varicocele I degree was 16.2±0.5 ml on the right and 16.3±0.5 ml on the left. According to ultrasound, the testicular volume in our patients with grade II varicocele was 15.8±0.8 ml on the right and 14.9±1.0 ml on the left. (Figure 3). In B-mode ultrasound, the bunched plexus veins appear as echonegative structures that are rectangular in the direct projection and round or oval in the transverse projection. Their clear localisation is not determined, more often the veins "envelope" the testis from all sides. In norm, the diameter of the left testicular vein is up to 25-3 mm, in varicocele it is the figure increases according to its degree.

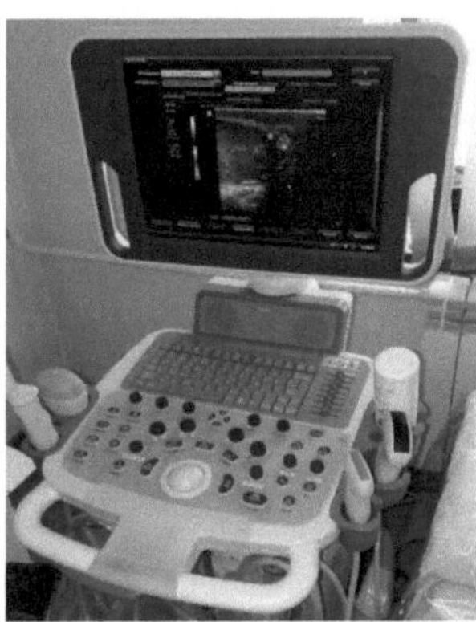

Figure 3. Mindray DC-N3 ultrasound scanner (China) with colour Doppler mapping.

We have shown the clarity of the results and the evaluation of the effectiveness of the performed examination on clinical examples. Ultrasound in varicocele in B-mode and Doppler provides volumetric information about the state of soft tissues, the degree of blood flow of the testicular tissue and its appendage.

Ultrasound of the scrotal organs in B-mode and with energy Doppler ultrasound to assess the state of tissues and the degree of blood flow in conjunction with spermogram indicators allows to diagnose not only the degree of varicocele, but also is a prognostic criterion for the diagnosis of primary infertility. That allows you to apply the most accurate treatment tactics or completely change the treatment process, thereby moving ultrasound from the category of additional methods of research in the main. Doppler mapping makes it possible to determine the degree of vascularisation of the scrotal organs, which allows the most reliable together with ultrasound data in B-mode to make an accurate diagnosis and choose an appropriate treatment tactic

Ultrasound examination of the scrotal organs with dopplerometry
Right testicle. Location: defined in the scrotum. Contours: smooth, clear. Testicular capsule: clear. Dimensions are not enlarged. Length 40 mm, thickness 35 mm, width 24 mm. Volume of the right testis: 17 cm^3. Echogenicity: typical. Echostructure: homogeneous. Structure of the mediastinum: preserved. Blood flow in the testis: preserved. Amount of fluid in the membranes: not enlarged. Testicular appendage: not enlarged. The veins of the cephalic plexus are 1.4 mm in clinostasis and 2 mm in orthostasis. At the height of the Valsalva test, pathological refluxes is undetectable.
Left testicle. Location: defined in the scrotum. Contours: smooth, clear. Testicular capsule: clear. Dimensions are not enlarged. Length 40 mm, thickness 31 mm, width 24 mm. Volume of the left testis: 16 cm^3. Echogenicity: typical. Echostructure: homogeneous. Mediastinal structure: preserved.
Testicular blood flow: preserved. Amount of fluid in the membranes: normal. Testicular appendage: not enlarged. The veins of the bunched plexus are 1.9 mm in clinostasis and 2.4 mm in orthostasis. At the height of the Valsalva test, pathological refluxes is undetectable.
Conclusion. No ultrasound signs of pathological changes were detected.

Scrotal echo-dopplerography.

In modern urology, ultrasound is widely used to examine men with reproductive disorders: testicles, appendages, vessels of the spermatic cord, prostate and seminal vesicles are examined, and in case of erectile dysfunction - the penis. USDG (ultrasound Dopplerography) is based on the Doppler effect, which consists in recording the measurement of the speed of reflected ultra sound waves from moving blood cells. Scrotal vascular Dopplerometry is a method of diagnosing the blood supply to the testicles. Spectral Doppler allows to distinguish between arterial and venous vessels, assessing the features of their blood flow (Table 2).

Table 2. Haemodynamic indices of blood flow in scrotal organs in norm (p ≤ 0.05)

Vessel	Linear blood flow velocity (LFV)	Index pulsativities (PI)	Resilience Index (RI)
Arteries seminal	0,114 ± 0,042	0,52 ± 0,020	0,59 ± 0,022
right channel			
Arteries of the vas deferens on the left	0,108 ± 0,036	0,5 ± 0,018	0,63 ± 0,013
Right testicular artery	0,118 ± 0,052	0,57 ± 0,02	0,61 ± 0,017
Left testicular artery	0,126 ± 0,027	0,45 ± 0,12	0,56 ± 0,017
Right parenchymatous testicular arteries	0,077 ± 0,012	0,67 ± 0,023	0,72 ± 0,011
Left parenchymatous testicular arteries	0,071 ± 0,031	0,45 ± 0,018	0,66 ± 0,024

In our studies, one of the tasks of preoperative examination of patients was to determine the nature of venous reflux into the spermatic cord plexus (haemodynamic type of varicocele) according to the classification of R.L.Coolsaet (1980).

1. Renotesticular reflux.

2. Ileotesticular reflux.

3. Combination of renotesticular reflux and ileotesticular reflux (mixed reflux).

To find out the haemodynamic type of varicocele, we used scrotal echo-dopplerography according to the method of E.B. Mazo et al. (1998), which is a modified method of C. Trombetta (1993). Trombetta (1993). Base The Department of Functional Diagnostics of the NF RRCEMP and City Hospital No. 1 were used for the study. The study was performed on a Mindray DC-N3 ultrasound scanner (China) with the possibility of colour Doppler mapping using a 7.5 MHz linear transducer in the seroscale echography mode, colour Doppler modes and in the pulsed-wave Doppler mode. Doppler techniques required setting the pulse repetition rate adequate for recording low-speed blood flow and using low-frequency filters. The value of the control volume was 1 mm. The study technology involved scanning the venous vessels of the bunched plexus at the level of the scrotal part of the spermatic cord and along the posterolateral surface of the testis (up to the projection of the lower pole of the testis and the tail of the appendage) in transverse, oblique transverse, longitudinal, and oblique longitudinal planes at rest and during the Valsalva test. The terminal portions of the testicular vein were visualised by translumbar and abdominal scanning. Colour Doppler imaging allowed to detect intra- and extra-ovarian arterial and venous blood flow and to assess the degree of vascularisation. Absolute (peak systolic blood flow velocity, end diastolic blood flow velocity, degree of venous return at the height of the Valsalva test) and relative (resistance index) quantitative indices characterising the state of the arterial and venous beds were determined by pulsed-wave Dopplerography.

The results of Doppler scanning of testicular veins allowed us to identify the following signs of haemodynamic types of varicocele according to R.L.Coolsaet (1980) . Absence of venous reflux - haemodynamic type 1 (corresponds to renospermatic reflux).

✓ Presence of venous reflux with a velocity equal to the initial velocity - haemodynamic type II (corresponds to ileospermatic reflux).

✓ The presence of venous reflux with a velocity significantly lower than the initial one - type III haemodynamic (corresponds to the combination of reno- and ileospermatic refluxes - mixed reflux).

The features of the echography techniques used were as follows: in adolescents, the normal diameter of renal veins was considered to be 3-4 mm.

Gradual enlargement of the left renal vein diameter compared to the right one and a decrease in the mean linear blood flow velocity (LFV) was considered an indirect sign of persistent venous renal hypertension. The symptoms of hypertension in the left renal vein in our study were considered to be an increase in its mean diameter compared with the right one by 2.0 ± 0.03 mm at rest and 3.0 ± 0.03 mm during the Valsalva exercise test.

On echo scanning, the veins of the spermatic cord were considered dilated if their internal diameter exceeded 3 mm and increased by more than 1 mm during the Valsalva stress test. When assessing the venous vessels of the plexus, when performing the Valsalva test in the supine position, a short-term (up to 1 sec.) retrograde blood flow into the veins of the plexus was detected in some patients on the left side. This short reflux was assessed as physiological. A prolonged retrograde blood flow wave lasting throughout the entire period of tension was considered pathological reflux. In the mode of colour Doppler mapping antegrade and retrograde blood flows were stained in different colours, which was also an objective evidence of blood reflux. Short isolated reflux into the upper segment of the testicular vein was also considered to be a physiological phenomenon; according to M.I. Pykov et al. (1999), it is associated with the absence of the vena cava mouth valves, and its cessation is associated with the closure of the vena cava wall valves.

In the study of the left renal vein to detect its compression and stenotic lesions, which was performed by echo-scanning in different Doppler modes, we used numerical criteria published in the literature (Table 2) (Fig. AMP). Detection of significant changes in the renal vein haemodynamics of com- pression stenotic character, as well as venous renal hypertension phenomena, requires the use of special methods and techniques of surgical treatment (vascular anastomosing operations), since, according to some authors, ligating operations in this case will not lead to improvement of testicular haemodynamics (Table 2). Such patients can be diagnosed as "secondary varicocele" ("varicocele with reno-testicular reflux and venous renal hypertension" - according to the classification of V.F.Bavilsky et al., which led to the exclusion of patients from the study. Moreover, Doppler detection of renal vein hemodynamic changes had a concomitant epidemiological aspect as a possible cause of varicocele development. (Table 3).

Table 3: Numerical criteria of Dopplerographic signs of renal vessel stenosis and compression in varicocele patients.

Stenosis criteria	"Aorto-mesen-tweezers."	Norma
Diameter renal vein at the site of stenosis, mm.	1,9 ± 1,0	2,3 ± 0,6
Diameter renal vein prestenotic of the section, mm.	10 ±2,0	7,2 ± 1,8
Max.velocity blood flow site	110,7 ±35,8	50,9±
stenosis,		27,9
cm/sec.		
Max. velocity blood flow in the prestenotic section, cm/sec.	14,2	18,6

Doppler studies in a number of patients revealed signs of renal vein compression in the aorto-mesenteric segment. All patients, as noted above, were subjected to urinalysis. It is known that the presence of protein in the urine in excess of 0.033 g/L, cylindruria, macro- and microhaematuria (the number of unchanged red blood cells over twenty in the field of view of the microscope) allows to suspect the presence of secondary renal nephropathy due to persistent compression changes in the renal vessels [65,66]. Taking into account the above mentioned Doppler criteria of compression lesions ("aorto-mesenteric pincer") and the absence of these urine changes, in such patients we assumed unexpressed compression and absence of persistent venous renal hypertension, which allowed us to include these patients in the study.

Ultrasound with Echo-Doppler allows to determine the following parameters of vein pathologies:

- Measurement thicknesses venous walls their increaseor decreased
- Detection of pathological changes in veins
- The nature of the vein valve lesions
- Degree of patency and diameter of the vessel lumen
- Presence of blood clots that obstruct blood flow
- Blood velocity.

Excretory or retrograde ureteroscopy (-graphy)

These radiological methods of examining the ureters, based on the kidney's ability to excrete specific radiopaque contrast agents, injected into the body,as a result which produces an image on the X-ray film. Image kidneys urinary and the urinary tract.as Urografin or urotrast is used as a radiopaque contrast agent. The drug is injected intravenously slowly (over 3 min) in excretory or urethrally in retrograde. The amount of contrast is based on the patient's weight. During ureteroscopy, no film is used and the progression of the contrast is observed on the monitor. A series of radiographs are performed in the following order: the first at 5-7th, the second at 12-15th, the third at 20-25 minutes, in case of delayed excretion of contrast agent, delayed radiographs are taken at 45 and 60 minutes. When analysing ureteroscopy (graphy), the functional state of the kidneys and patency of the ureters are assessed. It is imperative to have all emergency medical baggage on hand when performing this procedure.

Prostate specific antigen (PSA)

The introduction of PSA as a marker has revolutionised the diagnosis of prostate cancer (108). PSA is organ-specific, but is not considered cancer-specific, as it can be elevated in benign prostatic hyperplasia (BPH) and prostatitis and other non-malignant conditions. The PSA level as an independent indicator has a higher prognostic value than changes on PRI and TRUSI. There are no international standards for the measurement of PSA levels (110). PSA levels are considered to be "continuous" parameters, i.e. the higher the PSA level, the more likely it is to be cancer. Many men may present with RPV despite low blood PSA levels. B (Table 4). The rates of detection of RPF with a Gleason index ≥7 points (ISUP group 2) at low PSA levels are presented, which does not allow us to establish an optimal threshold for detecting nonpalpable but clinically significant RPF. The use of nomograms allows prediction of the detection of RPV.

Table 4: Cancer risk with low PSA levels

PSA levels, ng/ml	Cancer risk, % Risk Gleason index	≥ 7 points, %
0-0,5	6,6	0,8
0,6-1,0	10,1	1,0
1,1-2,0	17,0	2,0
2,1-3,0	23,9	4,6
3,1-4,0	26,9	6,7

PSA density is calculated by dividing the PSA level by the volume of the prostate as determined by TRUSI. The higher the PSA density, the more likely it is that the prostate cancer is clinically significant (see section 6.2.1 "Treatment of low-risk prostate cancer").PSA rise rate, PSA level doubling time There are two ways to measure changes in PSA levels over time:

1. PSA accrual rate, which is defined as the absolute annual increase in PSA (ng/ml/year) [113];
2. PSA doubling time, which expresses the exponential increase in PSA over time,

reflecting relative changes.

These two criteria may have prognostic value in patients who have undergone treatment for cancer. Nevertheless, their use in the diagnosis of prostate cancer is limited because of concomitant alterations (large GI volume, DGPH), unequal intervals between PSA measurements, and increases/decreases in PSA rise rate and doubling time over time. These indices do not provide additional prognostic information to PSA levels [116- 119]. The PSA ratio should be used with caution, as PSA levels may be affected by several methodological and clinical factors (instability of free PSA at room temperature and 4 °C, various conditions of analysis, concomitant large-sized GDM) [120].Nevertheless, this indicator can define the risk categories for BCP in men with total PSA levels between 4 and 10 ng/mL in the absence of changes on PRI. In a prospective multicentre study, BCP was detected at biopsy in 56% of men with c/o PSA < 0.1 and only 8% of men with c/o PSA > 0.25 ng/ml [121]. In addition, PSA c/o is of no clinical significance when total PSA is > 10 ng/ml and patients with previously diagnosed cancer are followed up.

PSA-3 is a prostate-specific, non-mRNA coding biomarker that is measured in urine sediment obtained after PG massage. A commercially available test, Progensa, is currently available. It is superior to total PSA and percentage free PSA in detecting RPJ in men with elevated PSA levels because it slightly but statistically significantly increases the area under the operating characteristic curve for a positive biopsy result. PSA-3 increases with increasing LV volume, but there are conflicting data on whether the Gleason index can predict PSA-3 levels, and its use as a monitoring tool for dynamic follow-up has not been confirmed. The main indication for PSA- 3 in urine may be an indication for repeat biopsy in men with a negative primary biopsy, but its cost-effectiveness has not yet been determined. The SelectMDX assay is based on mRNA biomarker isolation in urine. HOXC6 and DLX1 mRNA levels can determine the overall risk of detecting advanced and high-grade malignant prostate cancer on biopsy. According to published data, a number of biomarkers are more accurate than currently used prognostic parameters in differentiating aggressive and non-aggressive tumours.

CHAPTER III

DEVELOPMENT OF A CLASSIFICATION OF CYSTIC NEOPLASMS OF THE SCROTAL ORGANS

Diagnosis and treatment of fluid neoplasms of the scrotal organs is an urgent problem due to their frequency and the lack of a clear anatomo-topographical clinical classification and rational methods of diagnosis and surgical treatment, including simultaneous methods (Malyshev V.A. et al., 2015; Patil V. et al., 2015). The study of possibilities of surgical treatment of diseases of the organs of one or both halves of the scrotum by means of transmoshonojejunal access along the Wessling line is an urgent task in practical urology and andrology. In the emergency urology departments of the Sam. RRCEMP and Urology, 1-Samarkand City Hospital from 2021 to 2024, 138 patients with suspected fluid neoplasms of scrotal organs and prostate tumours were under our observation. Routine clinical examination methods as well as diaphanoscopy and ultrasound were performed. An attempt was made to develop a surgical classification of varieties of cystic neoplasms of the scrotal organs, and the surgical treatment of them was analysed, giving importance to simultaneous surgical interventions. 20 patients with unilateral, 30 patients with combined pathology of both halves of the scrotum and 23 patients with T4N0M0 prostate cancer were operated on. Operative treatment was performed by means of a single transmesoscrotal access along the Wesling line. When developing the classification of cystic neoplasms of the scrotal organs based on our materials, we took as a basis the classifications of Bosniak M A. (1997) for cystic neoplasms of the kidneys and Patil (1997). V. et al (2015) on "cystic fluid-filled lesions of the scrotum in adults".We decided to modify and adapt these classifications with respect to the scrotal organs, since by nature all cystic formations of different organs of the human body are almost identical. First, we present the classification of M.A. Bosniak (1986). According to this categorisation all varieties "cystic neoplasms of the kidneys are divided into the following forms (Fig.1) :

1. simple cyst - thin-walled, does not contain septa and calcifications;
2. benign cyst, containing several septa and calcifications;
3. cysts, with multiple septa;
4. doubtful cystic masses, have thickened walls and septa, benign or malignant;
5. established malignant masses, this includes also includes cystic cancer (Figure 4).

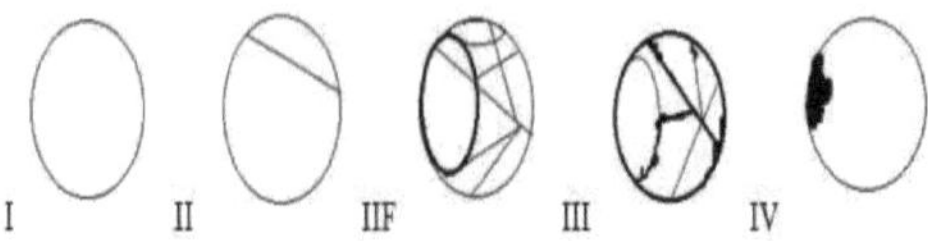

Figure 4. Renal cysts according to Bosniak classification (scheme).

Patil V. et al (2015) Classification:

1. Fluid in the scrotum: A. Congenital hydrocele; B. Seminal canal hydrocele; C. Acquired hydrocele; D. Haematocele; E. Pyocele; F. Lymphocele.
2. Testicular lesions: A. Whitecap cysts; B. Single or multiple cysts; C. Tubular ectasia; D. Epidermoid cysts; E. Testicular abscess; F. Intratesticular varicocele; H. Posttraumatic cysts.
3. Appendiceal cysts: A. Epididymal cysts; B. Spermatocele; C. Tubular ectasia of the testicular appendage; D. Testicular and testicular appendage cysts.
4. Groin and scrotal hernia.

In order to detect and substantiate each form of cystic neoplasm of the scrotal organs, it is of course necessary to carry out, in addition to routine examination methods, also thorough sonography, Doppler ultrasound, computed tomography, as well as histomorphological studies such as preoperative (puncture), intraoperative and postoperative (Bosniak M.A. 1997; Delyagin V.M. et al., 2014; Malyshev O.V. et al., 2015; Patil V.et al., 2015). As you know, any classification should be concise, low-word brief, but at the same time fully reflect the essence of the disease, to determine further therapeutic tactics.In constructing our classification, we were guided by these considerations for the purpose of simplification and convenience in the practical work of specialists. The order of individual nosological forms was observed by frequency, severity of course, difficulty of diagnosis, complications and complexity of treatment.(Table 5).

Table 5. Classification of cystic neoplasms of scrotal organs

№	Cystic category neoplasms	Nosological forms
1.	A simple benign cyst:	Testicular hydrocele, Funiculocele, Testicular cyst, A cyst of the spermatic cord, Cyst of the testicular of the testicular outgrowth, Testicular appendage cyst, Intrascrotal myoma.
2.	Simple benign complicated cyst:	Haematocele, Pyocele,
		Lymphocele, Spermatoceles, Epididymal cysts.
3.	Complicated cysts:	Testicular abscess, Post-traumatic cysts, Tubular ectasia of the testis, tubular ectasia of the testicular appendage, Epidermoid cysts.
4.	An inguinal hernia.	—
5.	Tumours of the scrotal organs .	—

As can be seen, all nosological forms are allocated into 5 groups, based on the nature of diagnosis and treatment:

I group - easily diagnosed, no active surveillance required;

II group - easy to diagnose, requires active surveillance;

III group-differential diagnosis difficult, dynamic observation, surgical treatment (minimally invasive, open, simultaneous);

IV group - diagnosis and treatment in conjunction with a surgeon ;

V group - diagnosis and treatment in conjunction with an oncologist.

When compiling this classification, we took into account common nosological forms studied and described in detail in the scientific literature (Bosniak M.A., 1997; Delyagin V.M. et al., 2014; Malyshev V.A. et al., 2015; Prokhorov A.V., 2016; Allazov S.A. et al., 2017; Okulov A.B. et al., 2018; Allazov I.S., 2021; Lelyavin K.B., 2022; Patil V. et al., 2015). Combined pathological conditions of the scrotal organs should be treated in an optimal simultaneous manner. We examined 202 patients with cystic neoplasms, which according to the given classification by nosological forms were distributed as follows (Table 6).

Table 6: Distribution of patients by nosological forms of cystic neoplasms of scrotal organs

Group	Nosological form	Abs.quantity	%
1	Simple benign cyst	75	37,1
2	Simple benign complicated cyst	42	20,7
3	Complicated cyst:	34	16,8
4	inguromastoid hernia	18	8,9
5	Tumours of the scrotal organs	10	4,5
6	Prostate tumours	23	11,3
Total		138	100,0

20 patients served as a control group, who were operated on in the traditional way on the side of the disease by lateral scrotal incisions. According to the data of objective examination and ultrasound examination, out of 20 patients with unilateral potology, 9 patients had cysts of the seminal canal, 5 had testicular cysts, 4 had epididymitis, 8 had orchitis, and 6 had orchoepididymitis. Out of 30 patients with bilateral potology, 16 had cysts of appendages of both testicles, 14 patients had cysts of the seminal canal. 8 patients were operated on for hydrocele on one side and testicular appendage cyst on the other side. In 23 patients with T4N0M0 prostate cancer, bilateral pulpectomy with subsequent treatment with antiandrogens was performed by the indicated access.

Clinical case 1. Patient S., 55 years old. He came in with complaints of pain and increased volume in the left side of the scrotum. On the basis of clinical and instrumental data, the diagnosis was made: "Left testicular appendage cyst" (Fig. 1.1), a scrototomy along the Wesling line was performed, and the left testicular appendage cyst was removed (Fig. 1.2,3). It should be noted that the postoperative scar formed at the Wessling line access looks like a scrotal suture. At re-examination of the patient in 1 and 3 months after the surgical intervention, a good cosmetic effect was noted, no recurrence of pathology was observed.

Clinical case 2. Patient N., 22 years old. He was admitted with complaints of pain in both halves of the scrotum, increased volume of the left half of the scrotum; On the basis of clinical and data, the diagnosis was made: "Left testicular sheath hydrocele, right testicular appendage cyst"; Scrototomy along the Wessling line, simultaneous performance of Winkelman's operation on the left and removal of the appendage cyst on the right were performed.

Clinical case 3. Patient N., 64 years old. Diagnosis: prostate cancer T3N1M0, osl: acute urinary retention. Operation: bilateral pulpectomy along the Wesling line, epicistostomy (Fig. 3.1,2,3,4.). This access is particularly convenient for performing bilateral orchiectomy or pulpectomy in advanced stages of prostate cancer during hormonal therapy of the underlying disease or for testicular tumours themselves. In addition, when suturing the scrotal skin, this access leaves an almost imperceptible postoperative scar resembling the Wessling line.

CHAPTER IV

TRADITIONAL SCROTOTOMIES AND SIMULTANEOUSSCROTA L ORGAN SURGERIES ALONG THE WESSLING LINE

As is known, frequent diseases of the external genital organs in men are malformations (midline separation of the sacs, underdevelopment, a- and hypoplasia of the testicles, testicular ectopia, cryptorchidism) (Kogan M.I.,2021), testicular torsion (Kalinina S.N.,et al.,2019), injuries (Nazarov T.H. et al., 2020), inflammatory diseases (epididymitis, orchitis, tuberculosis of the appendage and testis, brucellosis orchitis) (Bashembiev H.M. et al., 2010; Prokhorov A.V., 2016), fluid (testicular sheath dropsy, haematocele, funiculocele, spermatocele, varicocele) (Kapto A.A., 2016; Braz M.P. et al., 2013; Iacona F. etal., 2014; Rogue M. et al., 2018), tumours of the testis and its appendage.There is a special problem in relation to both, apparently healthy, testicles (bilateral pulp-or orchiectomy for prostate cancer) (Keshishev N.G. et al., 2010). In operations for the above-mentioned conditions, if unilateral, scrotal skin incisions are still made on the corresponding side of the disease or lesion. At the samc time, difficulties and difficulties arise in cases of a bilateral process requiring surgical intervention in both halves of the scrotum. Bilateral operative interventions on both testicles (orch-, pulpectomy) for prostate cancer are also problematic. Until now, many make incisions on both lateral surfaces of the scrotum, which is somehow traumatic, not cosmetic In this matter, it would be necessary to bear in mind the presence of the midline suture of the scrotum (Wesling's line), which is actually an extension of the white line of the abdomen on the scrotum (Leshenko I.G. et al., 2011; Allazov S.A. et al., 2018, 2020). The incision along this line is considered reasonable due to the simultaneous access through one incision to both halves of the scrotum and its organs, the so-called simultaneous operation (Allazov S.A. et al., 2018). The combination of pathologies of the organs of both halves of the scrotum, which leads to indications for simultaneous operations. Simultaneous operations are performed on different organs through a single access. Unlike multi-organ operations, they are performed on different organs simultaneously through different accesses. To perform simultaneous operations on the organs of both halves of the scrotum, the most convenient is the incision along the midline of the scrotum (raphe scroti), which is called by the name of the scientist who first described it - the Wesling line The Wesling line we conventionally divided into 4 parts (segments) anterior, at the bottom of the scrotum, posterior and perineal. Unlike all other authors, we decided to make the incision along the Wesling line in the posterior part, which does not affect the accessibility of the scrotal organs at all, but at the same time increases the cosmeticity of the postoperative scar, i.e. its visibility is absolutely lost, especially in the vertical position of the body. Cystic neoplasms of the scrotal organs have a peculiar clinical picture and require differentiated diagnosis, classification and appropriate treatment.The adapted classification of cystic neoplasms of the scrotal organs, based on the classification of Bosniak M.A. (1997) and Patil V. et al. (2015), covers the most frequent forms of diseases that are difficult to diagnose and require complex methods of treatment. Unilateral scrototomy or bilateral simultaneous surgical intervention through a single access along the Wessling line allows to perform several operations simultaneously on both halves of the scrotum and is the most optimal access for combined pathology of the scrotal organs (bilateral varicocele, testicular appendage cyst, hydrocele, lipoma of the scrotum, spermatic cord, etc.). This access is particularly suitable for performing bilateral orchiectomy or pulpectomy in advanced prostate cancer or testicular tumours. When suturing the scrotal skin, this access leaves an almost imperceptible postoperative scar resembling a Wessling line.It is quite common in clinical practice to encounter cases of combined pathologies of the organs of both halves of the scrotum, in connection with which there are indications for performing simultaneous operations. Simultaneous operations are performed on different organs through a single access. In contrast, in multi-organ operations, interventions on different organs are performed simultaneously through different accesses. To perform simultaneous operations on the organs of both halves of the scrotum, the most convenient is the incision along the midline of the scrotum (raphe scroti), which is called the Wesling's line after the name of the scientist who first described it. The study of the possibilities of surgical treatment of diseases of the organs of both halves of the scrotum by means of a single transmoshonojejunal access along the Wessling line is an urgent task in practical urology and andrology. From 2021 to 2024, we operated on 30 patients with combined pathology of both halves of the scrotum and 8 patients with prostate cancer T N M_{400}Surgical treatment was performed through a single transscrotal access using the Vesling line (J. Vesling (1598-1649) - professor of anatomy, surgery and botany at the University of Padua, who described the suture of the scrotum - raphe scroti, called the Vesling line. We conventionally divided Wesling's line into 4 parts (segments); anterior, at the bottom of the scrotum, posterior and perineal (Fig.5). In contrast to all other authors, we decided to make the Wesling incision posteriorly, which does not affect the accessibility of the scrotal organs at all, but at the same time increases the cosmeticity of the postoperative scar, i.e. its visibility is completely lost, especially in the vertical position of the body (Fig. 3).Patient O., 30 years old. He came in with complaints of pain in both halves of the scrotum, increased volume of the left half of the scrotum; On the basis of clinical and instrumental data, a diagnosis was made: "Left testicular sheath hydrocele; Winkelman's operation on the left side was performed by scrototomy. (Fig.7.1-7).

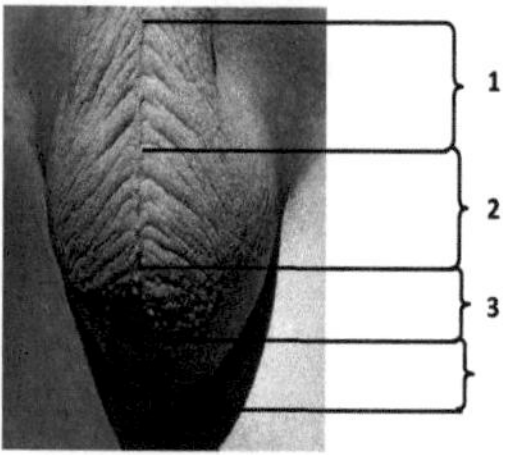

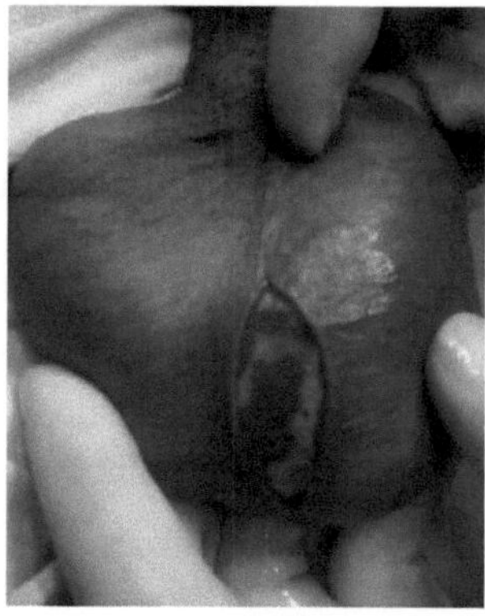

Figure 5. Raphe scroti - midline of the scrotum - Wessling's line: 1 anterior, 2 on the scrotal floor, 3 posterior, 4 perineal parts

Figure 6. Scrotal skin incision along the posterior Wesling's line

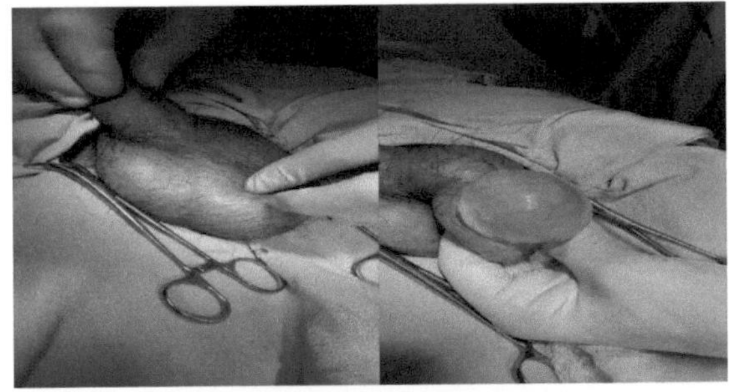

Fig 7. 1Pig 7.2

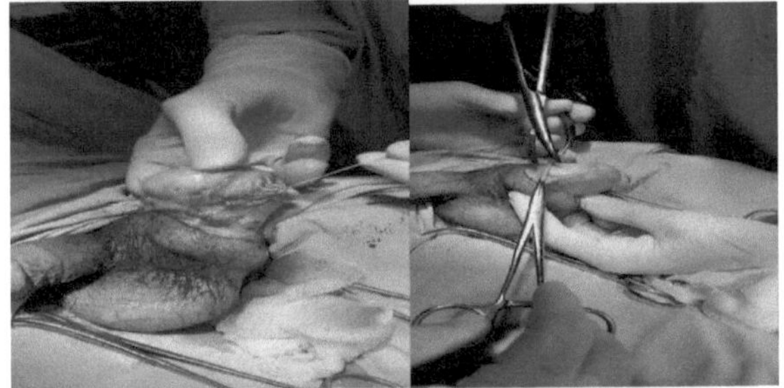

Figure 7.3Phase 7.4

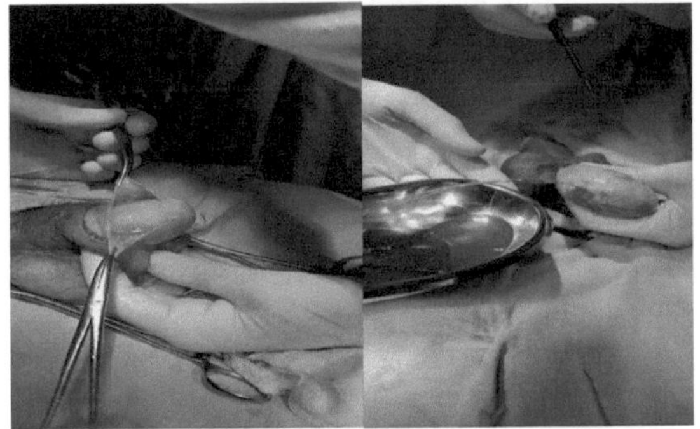

Figure 7.5Figure 7.6

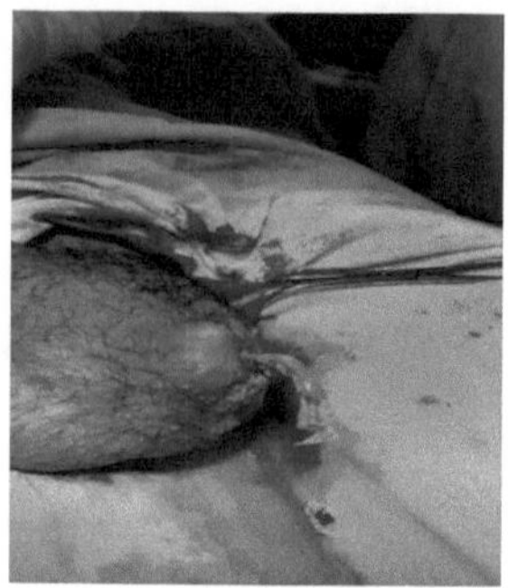

Fig 7.7

Fig.7 (7.1-7.7). Patient O. 30 years old. Scrototomy along the Wesling's line at the Various cystic neoplasms of the scrotal organs (description in text).

According to objective examination and ultrasonography, 13 patients had cysts of appendages of both testicles, 4 patients had a cyst of the spermatic cord and an appendage cyst of the opposite testis, 5 patients were operated on for hydrocele on one side and an appendage cyst on the other side. In 8 patients with prostate cancer T N M_{400} indicated bilateral pulpectomy with subsequent treatment with antiandrogens was performed. 20 patients served as the control group, in whom the operations were performed in the traditional way (incision) on the side of the disease by lateral scrotal incisions. (Fig. 4. 1,2,3,...). Patient N., 22 years old. He was admitted with complaints of pain in both halves of the scrotum, increased volume in the left half of the scrotum; On the basis of clinical and instrumental data, the diagnosis was made: "Left testicular sheath hydrocele, right testicular appendage cyst"; Scrototomy along the Wessling line, simultaneous Winkelman operation on the left and removal of the appendage cyst on the right were performed. (Fig. 8. 1,2,3,4,5,6)

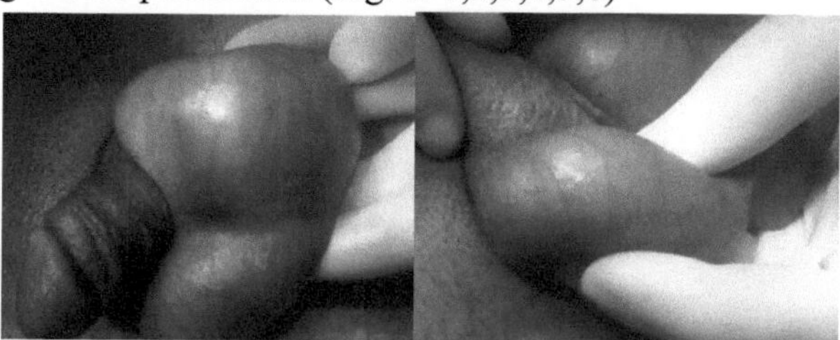

Fig.8.1 Fig.8.2.

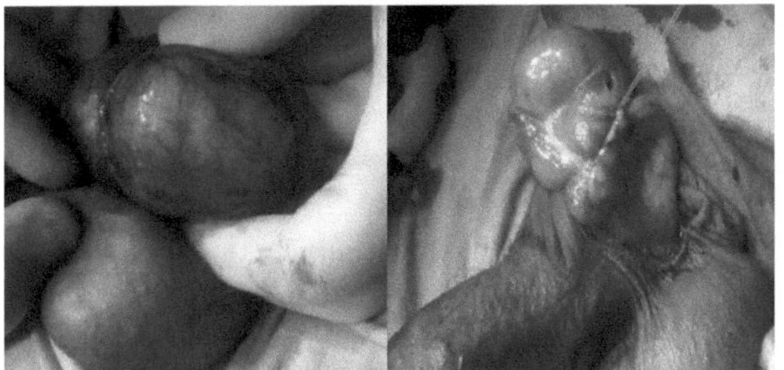

Figure 8. 3Figure 8.3

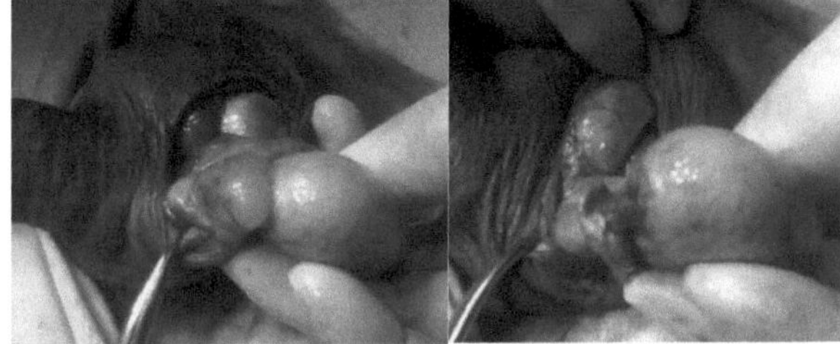

Figure 8.5.Figure 8.6.

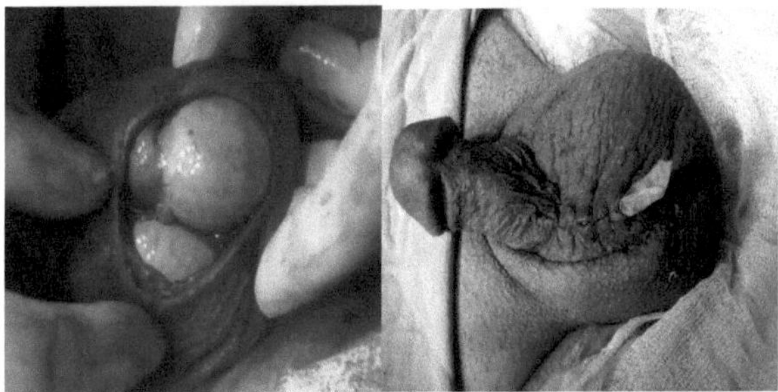

Fig. 8.7.Fig. 8.8

Fig.8 (8.1-8.8). Patient N. 22 years of age. Scrototomy along the Wessling line for various cystic neoplasms of the scrotal organs (description in text).

The use of the Wessling access allows simultaneous elimination of all existing problems through a single access to the scrotal organs. It should be noted that regardless of the method of suturing the scrotal skin at a single surgical access along the Wessling line, the formed postoperative scar looked like a scrotal suture. At the re-examination of the patients 1 and 3 months after the performed surgical intervention, a good cosmetic effect was noted, in none of the cases there was no recurrence of pathologies of either half of the scrotum. Thus Thus, it can be noted that surgical treatment through the Wesling access allows simultaneous multiple operations on both halves of the scrotum and is the most optimal access for combined pathology of the scrotal organs (testicular appendage cyst, hydrocele, bilateral pulpectomy, etc.). In addition, when suturing the scrotal skin, this access leaves behind an operative scar resembling raphe scrotum. Simultaneous surgical intervention through a single surgical access along the Wessling line allows several operations to be performed simultaneously on both sides of the scrotum and is the most optimal access for combined pathology of the scrotal organs (bilateral varicocele, testicular appendage cyst, hydrocele, lipoma of the scrotum, spermatic cord, etc.). This access is especially convenient for performing bilateral orchiectomy or pulpectomy in advanced stages of prostate cancer or testicular tumours. In addition, when suturing the scrotal skin, this access leaves an almost imperceptible postoperative scar resembling the Wessling line. As is known, frequent diseases of the external genitalia in men are malformations (midline separation of the sacs, underdevelopment, testicular a- and hypoplasia, testicular ectopia, cryptorchidism) (Kogan M.I.,2021), testicular torsion (Kalinina S.N.,et al.,2019), injuries (Nazarov T.H.,et al., 2020), inflammatory diseases (Voronik G.M., 2008; Bashembiev H.M., et al., 2010; Prokhorov A.V., 2015, 2016) (epididymitis, orchitis, tuberculosis of the appendage and testis, brucellosis orchitis), testicular hydrocele, haematocele, funiculocele, spermatocele, varicocele (Kapto A.A., 2016; Broz M.P. etal., 2013; Iacona F. etal., 2014; Rogue M. etal., 2018), tumours of the testis and its appendage. There is a special problem in relation to over both. seemingly healthy, testicles (bilateral pulpectomy for prostate cancer) (Keshishev N.G., et al. 2010). In operations on scrotal organs for different diseases, if they are unilateral scrotal skin incisions are usually made on the corresponding side of the disease or lesion (Nazarov T.H., et al., 2020; Kogan M.I., et al., 2021; Rogue M. et al., 2018), B At the same time, difficulties and complexities arise in cases of bilateral processes that require surgical intervention in both halves of the scrotum. Bilateral surgical interventions on both testicles (orch-, pulpectomy) for prostate cancer are also problematic. Many still make incisions on both sides of the scrotum, which is traumatic in one way or another. In operations for the above-mentioned conditions, if unilateral, scrotal skin incisions are usually made on the corresponding side of the disease or lesion. At the same time, difficulties and difficulties arise in cases of bilateral processes that require surgical intervention in both halves of the scrotum. Bilateral surgical interventions on both testicles (orch-, pulpectomy) in prostate cancer are also a problem. Many people still make incisions on both sides of the scrotum, which is traumatic in one way or another.In this matter, we should bear in mind the presence of the midline suture of the scrotum (Wesling's line), which is actually an extension of the white line of the abdomen to the scrotum (Leshenko I.G. et al., 2011; Allazov S.A. et al., 2015, 2019). The incision along this line is considered reasonable in order to access both halves of the scrotum and its organs, the so-called simultaneous surgery for various diseases (Allazov S.A. et al., 2018).Quite often in clinical practice there are cases of combined pathologies of the organs of both halves of the scrotum, and therefore there are indications for performing simultaneous operations. Simultaneous operations are performed on different organs through a single access. In contrast to multi-organ operations, interventions on different organs are performed simultaneously through different accesses. To perform simultaneous operations on the organs of both halves of the scrotum, the most convenient is the incision along the midline of the scrotum (raphe scroti), which is called by the name of the scientist who first described it - Wesling's line The study of the possibilities of surgical treatment of diseases of the organs of one or both halves of the scrotum by means of transmoshonojejunal access along the Wesling's line is an urgent task in practical urology and andrology. A midline Wesling incision (raphe scroti) is considered appropriate to access both halves of the scrotum and its organs, a so-called simultaneous operation for various diseases (Allazov S.A. et al., 2020, 2021). From 2021 to 2024 70 patients were observed. Among them 20 patients with unilateral, 30 patients with combined pathology of both halves of the scrotum and 18 patients with prostate cancer T4N0M0 were operated on. Surgical treatment was performed by means of a single transmesoscrotal access along the Wesling line. We conventionally divided the Wesling line into 4 parts: anterior, at the bottom of the scrotum, posterior and perineal. Unlike all other authors, we decided to make the incision along the Wessling line in the posterior part, which does not affect the accessibility of the scrotal organs at all, but at the same time increases the cosmeticity of the postoperative scar, i.e. its visibility is completely lost, especially in the vertical position of the body According to the data of objective examination and ultrasound examination, out of 70 patients with unilateral potology, 13 patients had cysts of the spermatic cord, 21 had testicular cysts, 15 had epididymitis, 4 had orchitis, and 6 had orchoepididymitis. Out of 30 patients, 13 patients had cysts of appendages of both testicles, 12 patients had a cyst of the spermatic cord and a cyst of the appendage of the opposite testicle, 8 patients were operated on for hydrocele on one side and a cyst of the appendage of the testicle on the other side. In 10 patients with T4N0M0 prostate cancer, bilateral pulpectomy with subsequent treatment with antiandrogens was performed by the indicated access. According to the data of objective examination and ultrasound examination out of 50 patients with unilateral potologia, 20 patients had cysts of seminal canal, 23 patients had testicular cysts, 17 patients had epididymitis, 8 patients had orchitis, 6 patients had orchoepididymitis. Out of 30 patients 16 patients had cysts of appendages of both testicles, 12 patients had cysts of seminal canal and cyst of appendage of opposite testicle, 8 patients were operated on for hydrocele on one side and cyst of appendage of testicle on the other side. In 10 patients with T4N0M0 prostate cancer a bilateral pulpectomy with subsequent treatment was performed by the indicated access with antiandrogens. This access is particularly suitable for bilateral orchiectomy or pulpectomy in advanced prostate cancer or testicular tumours. In addition, when suturing the scrotal skin, this access leaves an almost imperceptible postoperative scar resembling the Wessling line. In addition, when suturing the scrotal skin, this access leaves an almost imperceptible postoperative scar resembling the Wessling line. The use of the Wesling access allows simultaneous elimination of all existing problems through a midline access to the scrotal organs. It should be noted that the postoperative scar formed at the Wessling line access looked like a scrotal suture. At re-examination of the patients in 1 and 3 months after the surgical intervention a good cosmetic effect was noted, in none of the cases there was no recurrence of pathologies of any of the scrotal halves. Surgical treatment by means of surgical access along the Wessling line allows simultaneous several operations on both halves of the scrotum and is the most optimal access in case of combined pathology of the scrotal organs (testicular appendage cyst, hydrocele, bilateral pulpectomy, etc.). Moreover, when suturing the scrotal skin, this access leaves behind an operative scar resembling raphe scrotum. Scrototomy along the Wesling line was performed, Winkelman's operation on the left and appendiceal cyst removal on the right were performed simultaneously. Currently, the main method of prostate cancer treatment is antiandrogenic drug therapy. Due to the high cost of drugs and because of somatic contraindications, surgical castration is also widely used in clinical practice (Allazov S.A. et al., 2020; Allazov I.S. et al., 2021). The removal of both testicles in their entirety may lead to stress in some patients, which makes it necessary to develop medico-legal aspects of this problem. Orchiectomy helps to control the course of the disease and reduce its symptoms in about 90% of cases. Choice of treatment methods local and disseminated cancer and their sequence depend on the general condition of the patient and the sensitivity of the tumour to this or that treatment.

The essence of therapeutic measures is to maximally reduce the concentration of endogenous testosterone - the so-called androgen blockade. Orchidectomy is an effective method of reducing the main biological active androgen in the blood - testosterone, but has no effect on the production of adrenal androgens. Surgical castration is still considered the "gold standard" for anti-androgen therapy. Removal of the testes, which are the main source of androgens, results in a significant decrease in testosterone levels and causes a hypogonadal state, although negligible levels of testosterone remain (castration level). Bilateral orchiectomy is an easily performed surgical procedure that is performed under local anaesthesia and has virtually no complications. It is a quick (less than 12 hours) way to achieve castration testosterone levels.The standard castration level is considered to be <20 ng/dl. The main disadvantage of the method is the negative psychological effect. Most researchers confirm that the response of the body and the prostate can be determined by available methods: by objective tumour shrinkage, reduction of circulating PSA levels or simply by improvement of quality of life indicators such as pain, appetite, increased ability to work. In contrast to all other authors, we decided to make the Wesling incision for prostate cancer in 18 patients on the posterior surface of the scrotum. In patients with prostate cancer T N M_{400} bilateral pulpectomy with subsequent treatment with antiandrogens was performed using this access. This access is particularly suitable for performing bilateral orchiectomy or pulpectomy in advanced stages of prostate cancer or for tumours of the testicles themselves. In addition, when suturing the skin of the scrotum This access leaves an almost invisible postoperative scar resembling a Wesling line. Unilateral scrototomy or bilateral simultaneous surgical intervention through a single access along the Wessling line allows to perform several operations simultaneously on both halves of the scrotum and is the most optimal access for combined pathology of the scrotal organs (bilateral varicocele, testicular appendage cyst, hydrocele, lipoma of the scrotum, spermatic cord, etc.). This access is particularly suitable for performing bilateral orchiectomy or pulpectomy in advanced prostate cancer or testicular tumours. In addition, when suturing the scrotal skin, this access leaves an almost imperceptible postoperative scar, reminiscent of the Wessling line

CONCLUSION

Unilateral scrototomy or bilateral simultaneous surgery through a single Wesling access allows several operations to be performed simultaneously on both halves of the scrotum and is the most optimal access for combined scrotal pathology. This access is particularly convenient for performing bilateral orchiectomy or pulpectomy in advanced stages of prostate cancer or testicular tumours. In addition, when suturing the scrotal skin, this access leaves an almost imperceptible postoperative scar resembling the Wessling line.Simultaneous surgical intervention by Wesling suture in various pathological conditions of scrotal organs, contributes to the reduction of the duration of the operation time, shortening the time of patients' stay in hospital, rapid healing after the surgical wound.The Wessling incision on the posterior surface of the scrotum achieves complete cosmetic closure. A unilateral scrototomy or bilateral simultaneous surgery through a single Wessling access allows several operations to be performed simultaneously on both halves of the scrotum and is the most optimal access for combined scrotal pathology.This access is particularly suitable for performing bilateral orchiectomy or pulpectomy in advanced prostate cancer or testicular tumours. In addition, when suturing the scrotal skin, this access leaves a virtually invisible postoperative scar, resembling the Wessling line.

1. Surgical intervention using the Wessling suture for various pathological conditions of the scrotal organs contributes to the reduction of the duration of the operation time, shortening the time of patients' stay in hospital, rapid healing after the surgical wound.
2. By making a Wessling incision on the posterior surface of the scrotum, complete cosmeticisation is achieved.
3. In-depth examination of patients with diseases of the scrotal organs makes it clear that they are not sufficiently differentiated.
4. Accurate differential diagnosis with the use of orchidothermometry, USG and scrotoscopy contribute to pathogenic urgent surgical care and to avoid unnecessary orchiectomies.

5. In castration patients two accesses were operated, in both cases half of the scrotal skin forms rough postoperative scars with significant cosmetic defect, scrotal volume reduction is observed with the development of psychological dissatisfaction of the patient.
6. At pulpectomy with the Wesling access, regardless of the method of suturing

the scrotal skin, a postoperative scar is formed along the natural medial suture with a good cosmetic effect and preservation of the scrotal dimensions.
7. The advantages of single-stage Wessling line pulpectomy are less than bilateral trauma orchiectomy, the shorter duration of surgery is better with cosmetic efficiency and better psychological effect with short period of rehabilitation of patients.

PRACTICAL RECOMMENDATIONS

1. The clinical significance of the Wesling line, hitherto considered an anatomical concept, allows practising urologists to perform skin incisions along the Wesling line in surgical simultaneous treatment of the scrotal organs.
2. In oncological practice, bilateral orcho- or pulpectomy along the Wesling line is recommended for hormonal treatment of prostate cancer.
3. Performing the incision along the Wessling line creates conditions for saving surgical material, less traumatisation and cosmetic effect.

LITERATURE

1. Allazov SA, Allazov IS New concept of cystic neoplasms of scrotal organs (computed tomographic classification, simultaneous treatment) 2023; (150):34-40.
2. Allazov I.S. Optimisation of surgical access at simultaneous operations on scrotal organs. 2024.
3. Alyaev Y.G. Diseases of the prostate gland : a manual. - Moscow: Medforum, 2009. - 268 c. 10 Glybochko P.V., Alyaev Y.G. Practical urology. - Moscow: GEOTAR-Media, 2012. - 432 c.
4. Bashembnev H.M., Nazarkulov E.N., Akhmetkaliev A.J. Choice of treatment method for patients with acute inflammatory diseases of the appendage and testis. Journal of Almaty State Institute for Advanced Training of Physicians. (Bulletin of AGIUV) 2010; 3-4.
5. Batirov B.A., Gafarov R.R., Epidemiology of male urological pathology Uzbekistan through the prism of world statistics. Probl.biol. i med 2024 (152):310- 315
6. Belyaev A.L., Hodzhimetov T.A., Fozilov A.A. Vesicostomy in men with neurogenic dysfunction of lower urinary tract. XII Congress "Men's Health". Collection of theses. Kazan, 2016; 22.
7. Bratchikov OI, Hambaryan AA, Shumakova EA, Khmaruk AP, Trifonov EY Morphology of the bladder wall in patients with late-stage prostate adenoma // Mat. XII Russian Congress of Urologists, Moscow, 18-21 September 2012, P.
8. Bunatyan A.A., Mizikov V.M. Anaesthesiology: national manual. / edited by A.A. Bunatyan, V.M. Mizikov. Moscow: GEOTAR-Media, 2011. - 1104 c.
9. Gafarov R.R., Allazov H.S., Allazov I.S., Toshtemirov R.R. Operative access along the Wessling line at simultaneous operations on scrotal organs. Mater. 72nd Scientific and Practical Conf. of medical students and young scientists. Problems of modern medicine. Sam. 11-12 May 2018. Probl. biol. i med. 2018; 2-1 (101): 19.
10. Glybochko P.V., Alyaev Y.G., Grigorieva N.A. Urology. From symptoms to diagnosis and treatment: an illustrated guide. - Moscow: GEOTAR-Media, 2014. - 142 c.
11. Efremov. E.A. Kastrukin V., Melnik Ya.I., Simakov V,V., Yedoyan T A., Butov A. O. Results of the use of minimally invasive scrotal access performance of microsurgical varicocelectomy. Andrology 2019.,1:115- 119.
12. Efremov E.A. Melnik Y.I., Simakov V.V., Efremov E.A., Kastrikin Y.V.

Method of minimally invasive microsurgical varicocelectomy by scrotal access. Russian Federation patent for invention № 2 663 074 from 28.08.2018. Url://http://wwwl.fips.ru/wps/portal/IPS_Ru#15529833000276
13. Malignant neoplasms in Russia in 2007 (morbidity and mortality)/ edited by V. I. Chissov, V. V. Starinsky, G. V. Petrova. MOSCOW: FGU "P.A. Herzen MNIOI Rosmedtechnologii",2009.253 p.

14. Malignant neoplasms in Russia in 2011 (morbidity and mortality)/ edited by V. I. Chissov, V. V. Starinsky, G. V. Petrova. Moscow: P.A. Herzen MNIOM, 2013.289 p.
15. Kalinina S.N., Fesenko V.N., Burlaka O.O., Moshirev M.V., Alexandrov. M.S.. Tactics of treatment of patients with testicular torsion. Urological Vedomosti. 2019; 9 (1): 6-10.
16. Kogan M.I., Makarov A.G., Sisonov V.V., Kagantsov I.M., Orlov V.M. Results of the use of the original technique of testicular fixation at transsclerotal access in the surgery of cryptorchidism in children. Paediatric Urology Experimental and Clinical Urology 2021; 151-155.
17. Kapto A.A. Operative access along the Wesling line for varicocele. Andrology and Genital Surgery. 2016; 4: 44-48.
18. Clinical recommendations. Urology / ed. by N.A. Lopatkin. Moscow: GEOTAR-Media, 2007. 368 c.
19. Clinical staging of prostate cancer at its primary biopsy / S.B. Petrov, S.A. Rakul, A.V. Zhivov, R.A. Eloev, A.Y. Plekhanov, P.V. Kharchenko // Oncourology.2010. VOL.2. P.45-48.

20. Leshchenko I.G., Yakovlev O.G., Lazarev I.Yu., Shatokhina I.V. Planned simultaneous operations in urological patients of elderly and senile age, Urology. 2011; 4: 42-45.
21. Lysov N.A., Leshchenko I.G., Supilnikov A.A. Manual of abdominal surgery. - Samara: LLC "AZIMUT", 2016. - 436 c.
21. Nazarov T.H., Rychkov I.V., Trubnikova K.E., Lepekhina A.S., Khaknazarov H.U.. Organ-preserving operation at massive testicular smashing. Andrology and Genital Surgery. 2020; 5: 52-58.
22. Marchenkov V.E. Own clinical observations / O.G. Yakovlev, I.G. Leshchenko, V.V. Slivkin // C-multane urological operations in war veterans. - Samara: LLC "AZIMUT", 2012. - C. 125-126.
23.Matveev B.P.// Clinical Oncourology.- 2011.

24. Muslimov Sh.T. Comparative evaluation of laparoscopic and microsurgical varicocelectomy: Cand.kand.med.nauk. Moscow, 2013, 20 p.

25. Perepanova T.S., Komarova V.A. Peculiarities of functional disorders in pre-malignant hyperplasia hyperplasia prostate gland (pharmacoeconomic analysis)// Effective pharmacotherapy in urology.2007. No 2. C.12-22.
26. Pushkar D.Y. Radical prostatectomy. Moscow: MEDpress-Inform, 2004.

27. Manual of surgical diseases of the elderly / I.G. Leshchenko, R.A. Galkin. - 2nd ed., revision and add. - Samara: LLC "Ofort", 2016. - 494 c.

28. Urology, national guide / ed. by Acad. RAMS N.A.Lopatkin. - Moscow: GEOTAR-Media, 2009. - 1024 c.

29. Prokhorov. A.V. Abscess of the scrotum. Perm Medical Journal 2016: 33 (3):102-109.
29. Urology: national manual. / ed. by N.A. Lopatkin. Moscow: GEOTAR-Media, 2009. 1024 c.

30. Chechenin M. G., Robustov V. V. Urgent transurethral electroresection for acute urinary retention in patients with adenoma and prostate cancer // Scientific Conference of Urologists, Uzbekistan.1981. C.69-70
31. Yakovlev O.G., Leshchenko I.G., Slivkin V.V. Simultaneous urological operations in war veterans. - Sara Mara: LLC "AZIMUT", 2012 . - 163 c.
32. Yakovlev O.G., Leshchenko I.G., Slivkin V.V. Simultaneous urological operations in war veterans. Samara: AZIMUT, 2012.
33. Braz M.P., Martins F., Castagnaro A. et al. Trans-Scrotum "En Bloc "Varicocele Ressection: A New Approach That Prevents Post Operative Hydrocele. Pediatric Urology Fall Congress, 2013. Las Vegas, Nevada, Available at: http fallcongress.spuonline.orgabstract 2013; 39.
34. Bozhedomov V.A., Lipatova N.A., Alexeev R.A. et al. The role of the antisperm antibodies in male infertility assessment after microsurgical varicocelectomy. Andrology. 2014;2:847-855.
35. Bozhedomov V., Alexandrova M., Sukhikh G. et al. The role of the antisperm antibodies in male infertility assessment after microsurgical varicocelectomy. Andrology. 2014;2(6):847-855.
36. Baazeem A., Boman J.M., Libman et al. Microsurgical varicocelectomy for infertile men with oligospermia: Differential effect of bilateral and unilateral varicocele on pregnancy outcomes. BJU International, 2009;104(4): 524-528.
37. Baazeem A., Belzile E., Ciampi A. et al. Varicocele and male factor infertility treatment: a new meta-analysis and review of the role of varicocele repair. Eur Urol. 2011;60(4):796-808.
38. Barratt C.L.R., Bjurndahl L., De Jonge C.J. et al. The diagnosis of male

infertility: an analysis of the evidence to support the development of global WHO guidance- challenges and future research opportunities. Hum Reprod Update. 2017;23(6):660- 680.
39. Borruto FA, Impellizzeri P, Antonuccio P. Laparoscopic vs. open varicocelectomy in children and adolescents: review of the recent literature and meta-analysis. Journal of Pediatric Surgery. 2010; 45(12): 2464-9.
40. Barone JG, Johnson K, Sterling M, Ankem MK. Laparoendoscopic single-site varicocele repair in adolescents - initial experience at a single institution. Journal of Endourology. 2011; 25: 1605-8.
41.Cayan S, Shavkat S, Kadioglu A. Treatment of palpable varicocele in Infertile men: a meta-analysis to define the best technique .JAndrol 2009;30(1):33-40. Doi:10.2164\jandrol.108.005967
42. Cayan S, Şahin S, Akbay E. Paternity Rates and Time to Conception in Adolescents with Varicocele Undergoing Microsurgical Varicocele Repair vs Observation Only: A Single Institution Experience with 408 Patients. J Urol. 2017;198(1):195-201.
43. Coban S, Keles I, Biyik I, Guzelsoy M, Turkoglu AR, OcakN. Does varicocele correction lead to normalisation of preoperatively elevated mean platelet volume levels? Canadian Urologic Associaction Journal. 2015; 9: 5-9.
44.Comhaire F. Clinical andrology: from evidence to ethics. The "E" quintet in clinical andrology. Hum Reprod. 2000;15(10):2067–2071.
45.Cantoro U., Catanzariti F., Lacetera V. et al. Percentage change of FSH value: a new variable to predict the seminal outcome after varicocelectomy. Andrologia. 2015;47:412-416.
46. Demir Ö, Temizkan AK. Spontaneous Rupture Of Varicocele Due To Strain Defecation. Dokuz Eylül Üniversitesi Tıp Fakültesi Derg. 2010;24: 33-6.
47. Deniz Bolat, Bulent Gunlusoy,MD, , Serkan Yarimoglu, MD, et al. Isolated thrombosis of right spermatic vein with underlying factor V Leiden mutation. Can Urol Assoc J 2016; 10(9-10): E324-E327.
48. Dada R., Venkatesh S., Kumar K.et al. Re: Decreased sperm DNA fragmentation after surgical varicocelectomy is associated with increased pregnancy rate: M. Smit,
J.C. Romijn, M.W. Wildhagen, J.L. Veldhoven, RF. Weber and G.R. Dohle. J Urol. 2010;183:270-274. J Urol. 2010; 184: 1577 (author reply 1578).
49. Ding H., Tian J., Du W. et al. Open non-microsurgical, laparoscopic or open microsurgical varicocelectomy for male infertility: a meta-analysis of randomised controlled trials. BJU Int. 2012;110(10):1536–1542.

50. Dohle GR, Diemer T, Givercman A. Male infertility. European Association of Urology Guidelines. 2011; 32-4.
51. Eid R, Radad K, Al-Shraim M. Ultrastructural changes of smooth muscles in varicocele veins. Ultrastructural Pathology. 2012; 36(4): 201-6.
52. Elzanaty S. Varicocele repair in non-obstructive azoospermic men: diagnostic value of testicular biopsy - a meta-analysis. Scandinavian Journal of Urology. 2014; 48(6): 494-8.
53. El Hennawy HM, Abuzour ME, Bedair ESM. Surgical management of spontaneously thrombosed extratesticular varicocele presented with irreducible inguinal swelling: a case report. Eur. J Surg Sci. 2010;1(3):99-101.
54. Goren M.R., Erbay G., Ozer C. et al. Can We Predict the Outcome of Varicocelectomy Based on the Duration of Venous Reflux? Urology. 2016;88:81-86.
55. Garg H, Kumar R. An update on the role of medical treatment including antioxidant therapy in varicocele. Asian Journal of Andrology. 2016; 18, 222-228.
56. Gosalvez J., Lopez-Fernandez C., Fernandez J.L.. Sperm chromatin dispersion test: technical aspects and clinical applications. Biological and Clinical Applications in MaleInfertility and Assisted Reproduction. 2011. Springer: 151-170.
57. Iacono F., Ruffo A.,Prezioso D. et al. Treatment of bilateral varicocele and other scrotal comorbidities using a single scrotal access: our experience on 34 patients. Biomedes Int. 2014: 403603. DOI: 10.1155/2014/403603.
58. Johnson D., Harnisch B., Zganjar A. et al. Mp74-13 Predictors of success after microscopic subinguinal varicocelectomy. J Urol. 2015;193(4):e944.
59. Jensen C.F.S., Sstergren P., Dupree J.M. et al. Varicocele and male infertility. Nat Rev Urol. 2017; 14(9): 523-533.
60. Roque M. Esteves SC. Effect of varicocele repair on sperm DNA fragmentation: a review. Int Urol Nephrol 2018; 5(4): 583 603. Doi:10.1007/s11255-018-1839-4.
61. Zampieri N., Zampieri G., Antonello L., Camoglio F.S. Trans-scrotal varicocelectomy in adolescents: Clinical and surgical outcomes. J Pediatr Surg 2014;49:583-5.
62. Çoban S, Keleş I, Biyik I, Güzelsoy M, Türkoğlu AR, Özgünay T et al. Is there any relationship between mean platelet volume and varicocele? Andrologia. 2015; 47: 37- 41.

63. Chen Q, Zhong L, Wu S, Sun Y, Ju G, Sun J. Laparoscopic varicocelectomy with single incision in children. Laparoscopic Urology. 2015; 12(6): 2400-3.

64. Vozianov S.O., Ishmuradov B.T.Androgen deprivation theeapy for prostate canser. LAD LAMBERT Academik Publishing. 2023.

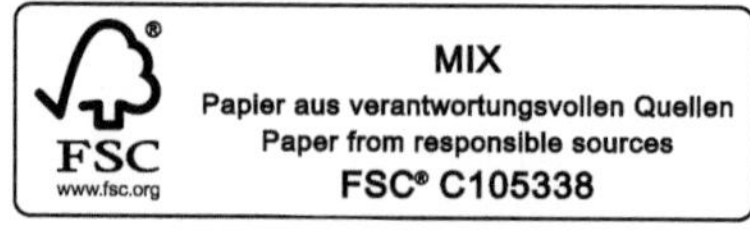

Printed by Books on Demand GmbH, Norderstedt / Germany